My 28 Day Keto Journey

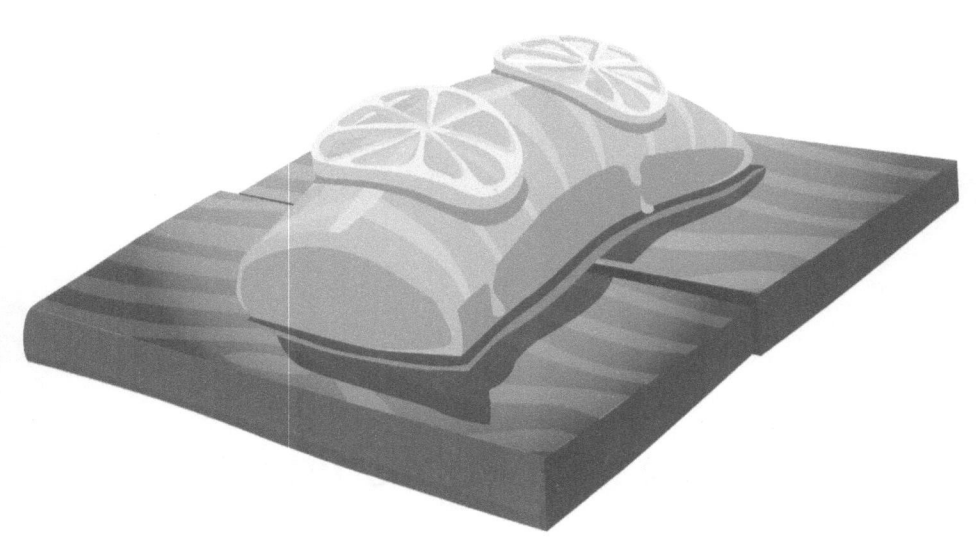

Advanta Publishing

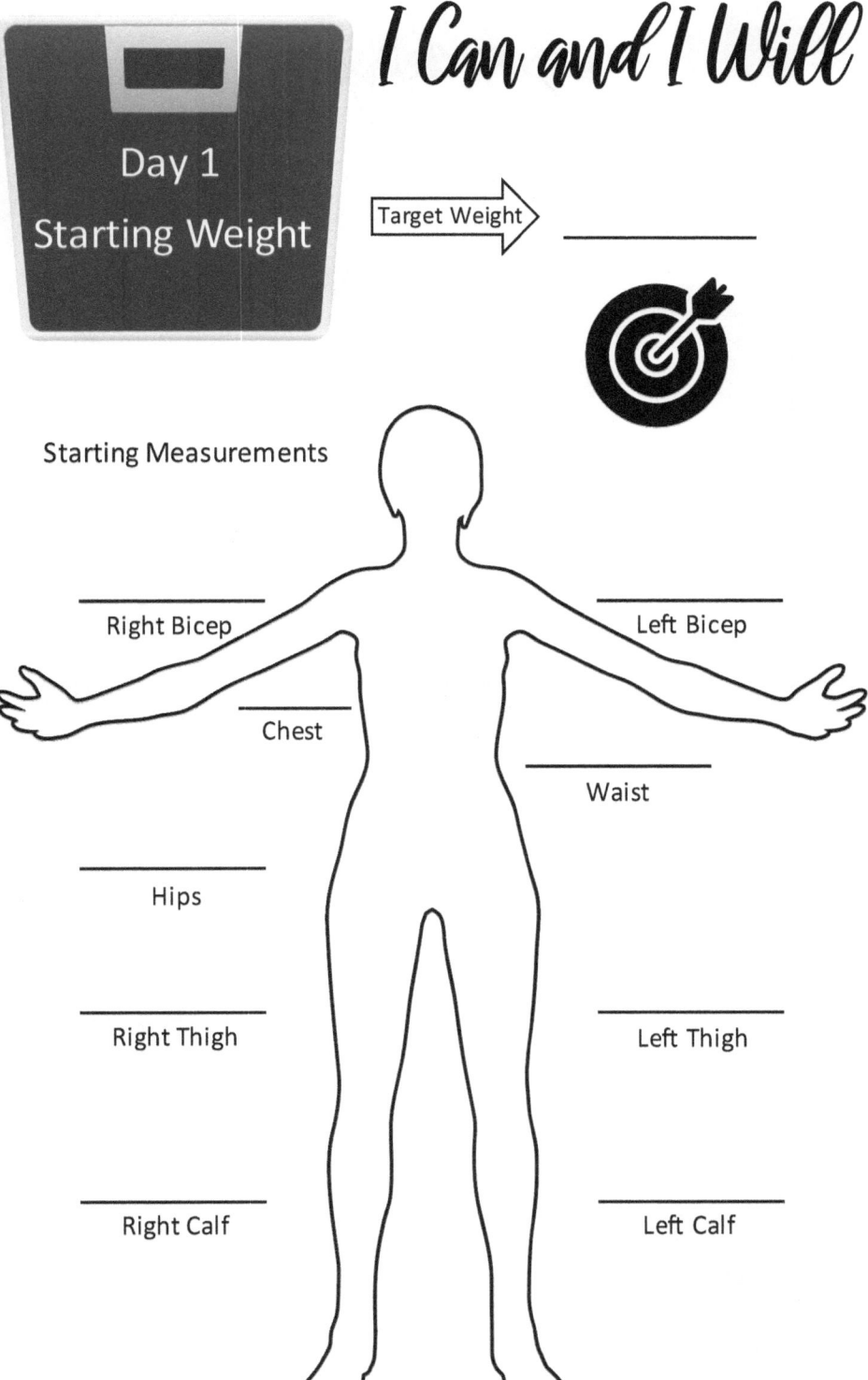

I Can and I Will

Day 1
Starting Weight

Target Weight

Starting Measurements

Right Bicep

Left Bicep

Chest

Waist

Hips

Right Thigh

Left Thigh

Right Calf

Left Calf

Before

4"x6"

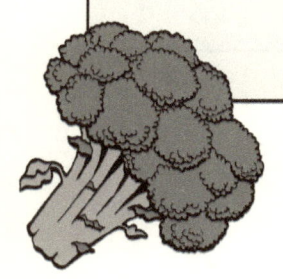

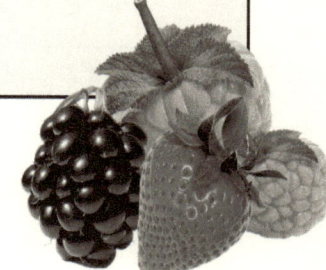

Questions To Ask Myself

Why am I starting the Keto lifestyle?

_____

_____

_____

_____

What's my end goal?

_____

_____

_____

_____

Do I have a weight loss mindset?

_____

_____

_____

_____

Who can I count on for support?

_____

_____

_____

_____

Day 1 – 7

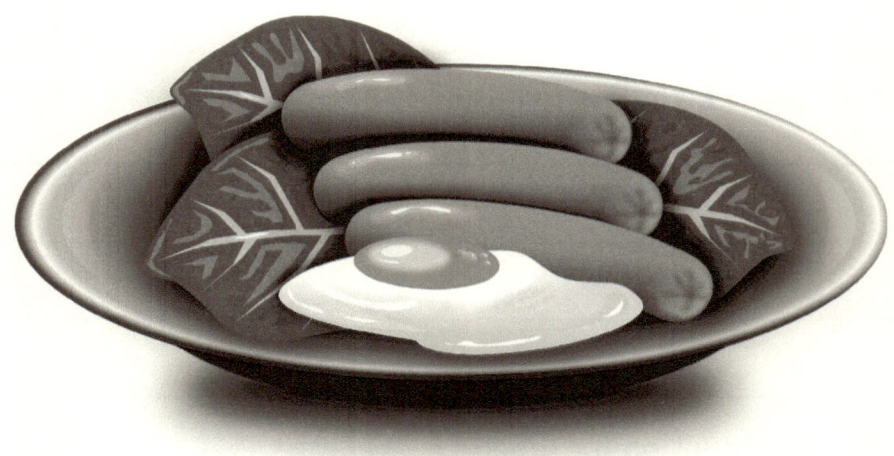

Meal Planner

Day 1 – 7

Day 1	Breakfast: Lunch: Dinner:
Day 2	Breakfast: Lunch: Dinner:
Day 3	Breakfast: Lunch: Dinner:
Day 4	Breakfast: Lunch: Dinner:
Day 5	Breakfast: Lunch: Dinner:
Day 6	Breakfast: Lunch: Dinner:
Day 7	Breakfast: Lunch: Dinner:
Snacks	

Shopping List

MEAT & FISH	DAIRY	VEGETABLES
Bacon	Heavy Cream	Broccoli
Ground Beef	Full Fat Yogurt	Cauliflower
Chicken	Eggs	Cabbage
Cold Cuts	Butter	Cucumber
Pork	Ghee	Eggplant
Lamb	Sour Cream	Bell Pepper
Organ Meats	Cream Cheese	Asparagus
Duck	Full Fat Cheeses	Salad Mix
Steak	**PANTRY**	Spaghetti Squash
Sausage	Pork Rinds	Zuchinni
Shrimp	Almond Milk	Onions
Salmon	Coconut Milk	Garlic
Tuna	Coffee	Celery
FATS & OILS	Himalayan Pink Salt	**FRUITS**
Olive Oil	Mustard	Avocados
Avocado Oil	90% Dark Chocolate	Blueberries
Sesame Oil	Almond Flour	Blackberries
MCT Oil	Coconut Flour	Raspberries
Lard	Bone Broth	Strawberries
Cocoa Butter	Xanthan Gum	Lemons
Coconut Oil	Erythritol	Limes
Nut Butters	Monkfruit	Nuts & Seeds

Shopping List

Day 1 – 7

MEAT & FISH	DAIRY	VEGETABLES
	PANTRY	
FATS & OILS		FRUITS

Habit Tracker

HABIT	1	2	3	4	5	6	7	REWARD

Mood Tracker

DAY	MOOD					WHY?
1	☺	☻	☹	☹	☹	
2	☺	☻	☹	☹	☹	
3	☺	☻	☹	☹	☹	
4	☺	☻	☹	☹	☹	
5	☺	☻	☹	☹	☹	
6	☺	☻	☹	☹	☹	
7	☺	☻	☹	☹	☹	

 Only I can change my life!
No one can do it for me.

Exercise Tracker

Day 1	Day 2	Day 3
Cardio ○ Weights ○	Cardio ○ Weights ○	Cardio ○ Weights ○

Day 4	Day 5	Day 6
Cardio ○ Weights ○	Cardio ○ Weights ○	Cardio ○ Weights ○

Day 7	Day	Calories Burned
	1	
	2	
	3	
	4	
	5	
Cardio ○	6	
Weights ○	7	

Day 1 Food Tracker

Date: _____

MON TUE WED THU FRI SAT SUN

Daily Target						
Breakfast	Calories	Fat	Protein	Carbs	Fiber	Net Carbs
Total:						
Lunch	Calories	Fat	Protein	Carbs	Fiber	Net Carbs
Total:						
Dinner	Calories	Fat	Protein	Carbs	Fiber	Net Carbs
Total:						
Snacks	Calories	Fat	Protein	Carbs	Fiber	Net Carbs
Total:						
Daily Total						

Ketosis: Y/N   Intermittent Fasting: From _____am/pm - To_____am/pm

How'd I do?

Day 2   Food Tracker

Daily Target						
Breakfast	Calories	Fat	Protein	Carbs	Fiber	Net Carbs
Total:						
Lunch	Calories	Fat	Protein	Carbs	Fiber	Net Carbs
Total:						
Dinner	Calories	Fat	Protein	Carbs	Fiber	Net Carbs
Total:						
Snacks	Calories	Fat	Protein	Carbs	Fiber	Net Carbs
Total:						
Daily Total						

Ketosis: Y/N   Intermittent Fasting: From _____am/pm - To_____am/pm

How'd I do?

Day 3 Food Tracker

Daily Target						
Breakfast	Calories	Fat	Protein	Carbs	Fiber	Net Carbs
Total:						
Lunch	Calories	Fat	Protein	Carbs	Fiber	Net Carbs
Total:						
Dinner	Calories	Fat	Protein	Carbs	Fiber	Net Carbs
Total:						
Snacks	Calories	Fat	Protein	Carbs	Fiber	Net Carbs
Total:						
Daily Total						

Ketosis: Y/N   Intermittent Fasting: From _____am/pm - To_____am/pm

How'd I do?

Day 4   Food Tracker

Date: _____
MON TUE WED THU FRI SAT SUN

Daily Target						
Breakfast	Calories	Fat	Protein	Carbs	Fiber	Net Carbs
Total:						
Lunch	Calories	Fat	Protein	Carbs	Fiber	Net Carbs
Total:						
Dinner	Calories	Fat	Protein	Carbs	Fiber	Net Carbs
Total:						
Snacks	Calories	Fat	Protein	Carbs	Fiber	Net Carbs
Total:						
Daily Total						

Ketosis: Y/N   Intermittent Fasting: From _____am/pm - To_____am/pm

How'd I do?

Day 5　　Food Tracker

Daily Target						

Breakfast	Calories	Fat	Protein	Carbs	Fiber	Net Carbs
Total:						

Lunch	Calories	Fat	Protein	Carbs	Fiber	Net Carbs
Total:						

Dinner	Calories	Fat	Protein	Carbs	Fiber	Net Carbs
Total:						

Snacks	Calories	Fat	Protein	Carbs	Fiber	Net Carbs
Total:						

Daily Total						

Ketosis: Y/N　　Intermittent Fasting: From _____am/pm - To_____am/pm

How'd I do?

Day 6   Food Tracker

Date: _____
MON TUE WED THU FRI SAT SUN

Daily Target						
Breakfast	Calories	Fat	Protein	Carbs	Fiber	Net Carbs
Total:						
Lunch	Calories	Fat	Protein	Carbs	Fiber	Net Carbs
Total:						
Dinner	Calories	Fat	Protein	Carbs	Fiber	Net Carbs
Total:						
Snacks	Calories	Fat	Protein	Carbs	Fiber	Net Carbs
Total:						
Daily Total						

Ketosis: Y/N   Intermittent Fasting: From _____am/pm - To_____am/pm

How'd I do?

Day 7   *Food Tracker*

Date: _____
MON TUE WED THU FRI SAT SUN

Daily Target						
Breakfast	Calories	Fat	Protein	Carbs	Fiber	Net Carbs
Total:						
Lunch	Calories	Fat	Protein	Carbs	Fiber	Net Carbs
Total:						
Dinner	Calories	Fat	Protein	Carbs	Fiber	Net Carbs
Total:						
Snacks	Calories	Fat	Protein	Carbs	Fiber	Net Carbs
Total:						
Daily Total						

Ketosis: Y/N   Intermittent Fasting: From _____am/pm - To_____am/pm

How'd I do?

After 7 Days

4"x6"

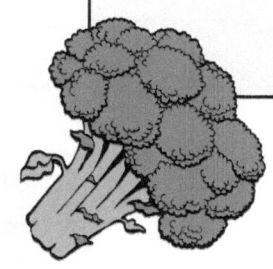

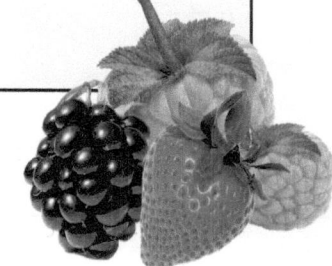

Questions To Ask Myself

Why am I starting the Keto lifestyle?

_____

_____

_____

_____

What's my end goal?

_____

_____

_____

_____

Do I have a weight loss mindset?

_____

_____

_____

_____

Who can I count on for support?

_____

_____

_____

_____

Day 8 – 14

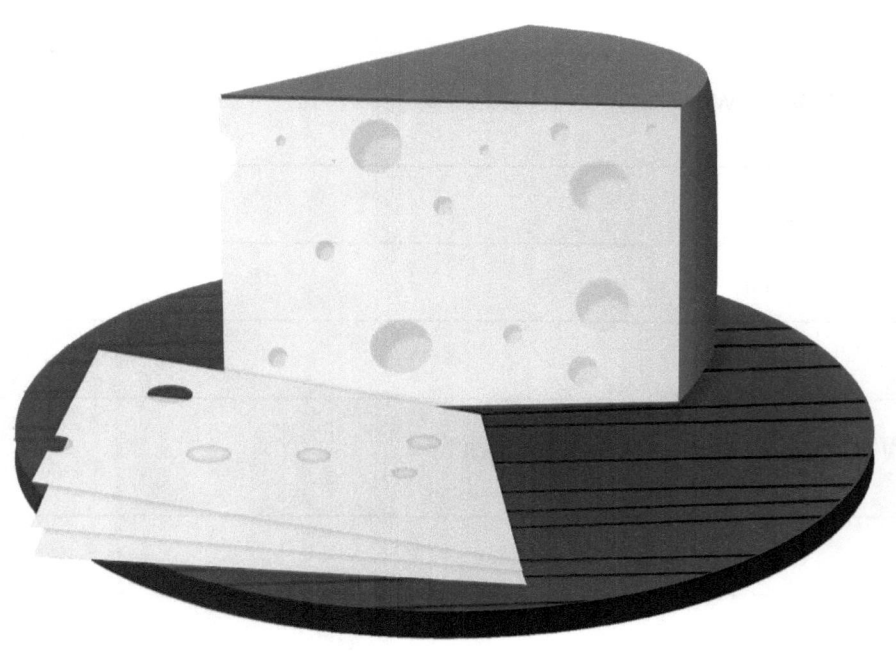

Meal Planner

Day 8	Breakfast: Lunch: Dinner:
Day 9	Breakfast: Lunch: Dinner:
Day 10	Breakfast: Lunch: Dinner:
Day 11	Breakfast: Lunch: Dinner:
Day 12	Breakfast: Lunch: Dinner:
Day 13	Breakfast: Lunch: Dinner:
Day 14	Breakfast: Lunch: Dinner:
Snacks	

Shopping List

MEAT & FISH	DAIRY	VEGETABLES
Bacon	Heavy Cream	Broccoli
Ground Beef	Full Fat Yogurt	Cauliflower
Chicken	Eggs	Cabbage
Cold Cuts	Butter	Cucumber
Pork	Ghee	Eggplant
Lamb	Sour Cream	Bell Pepper
Organ Meats	Cream Cheese	Asparagus
Duck	Full Fat Cheeses	Salad Mix
Steak	**PANTRY**	Spaghetti Squash
Sausage	Pork Rinds	Zuchinni
Shrimp	Almond Milk	Onions
Salmon	Coconut Milk	Garlic
Tuna	Coffee	Celery
FATS & OILS	Himalayan Pink Salt	**FRUITS**
Olive Oil	Mustard	Avocados
Avocado Oil	90% Dark Chocolate	Blueberries
Sesame Oil	Almond Flour	Blackberries
MCT Oil	Coconut Flour	Raspberries
Lard	Bone Broth	Strawberries
Cocoa Butter	Xanthan Gum	Lemons
Coconut Oil	Erythritol	Limes
Nut Butters	Monkfruit	Nuts & Seeds

Shopping List

MEAT & FISH	DAIRY	VEGETABLES
	PANTRY	
FATS & OILS		**FRUITS**

Habit Tracker

HABIT	8	9	10	11	12	13	14	REWARD

Mood Tracker

DAY	MOOD					WHY?
8	☺	☻	☹	☹	☹	
9	☺	☻	☹	☹	☹	
10	☺	☻	☹	☹	☹	
11	☺	☻	☹	☹	☹	
12	☺	☻	☹	☹	☹	
13	☺	☻	☹	☹	☹	
14	☺	☻	☹	☹	☹	

 *If you are tired of starting over Stop giving up!*

Exercise Tracker

Day 8	Day 9	Day 10
Cardio ◯ Weights ◯	Cardio ◯ Weights ◯	Cardio ◯ Weights ◯

Day 11	Day 12	Day 13
Cardio ◯ Weights ◯	Cardio ◯ Weights ◯	Cardio ◯ Weights ◯

Day 14	Day	Calories Burned
	8	
	9	
	10	
	11	
	12	
	13	
Cardio ◯ Weights ◯	14	

Day 8 *Food Tracker*

Daily Target						

Breakfast	Calories	Fat	Protein	Carbs	Fiber	Net Carbs
Total:						

Lunch	Calories	Fat	Protein	Carbs	Fiber	Net Carbs
Total:						

Dinner	Calories	Fat	Protein	Carbs	Fiber	Net Carbs
Total:						

Snacks	Calories	Fat	Protein	Carbs	Fiber	Net Carbs
Total:						

Daily Total						

Ketosis: Y/N   Intermittent Fasting: From _____am/pm - To_____am/pm

How'd I do?

Day 9   Food Tracker

Date: _____
MON TUE WED THU FRI SAT SUN

Daily Target						
Breakfast	Calories	Fat	Protein	Carbs	Fiber	Net Carbs
Total:						
Lunch	Calories	Fat	Protein	Carbs	Fiber	Net Carbs
Total:						
Dinner	Calories	Fat	Protein	Carbs	Fiber	Net Carbs
Total:						
Snacks	Calories	Fat	Protein	Carbs	Fiber	Net Carbs
Total:						
Daily Total						

Ketosis: Y/N   Intermittent Fasting: From _____am/pm - To_____am/pm

How'd I do?

Day 10   Food Tracker

Date: _____

Daily Target						
Breakfast	Calories	Fat	Protein	Carbs	Fiber	Net Carbs
Total:						
Lunch	Calories	Fat	Protein	Carbs	Fiber	Net Carbs
Total:						
Dinner	Calories	Fat	Protein	Carbs	Fiber	Net Carbs
Total:						
Snacks	Calories	Fat	Protein	Carbs	Fiber	Net Carbs
Total:						
Daily Total						

Ketosis: Y/N   Intermittent Fasting: From _____am/pm - To_____am/pm

How'd I do?

Day 11   Food Tracker

Date: _____

MON TUE WED THU FRI SAT SUN

Daily Target						
Breakfast	Calories	Fat	Protein	Carbs	Fiber	Net Carbs
Total:						
Lunch	Calories	Fat	Protein	Carbs	Fiber	Net Carbs
Total:						
Dinner	Calories	Fat	Protein	Carbs	Fiber	Net Carbs
Total:						
Snacks	Calories	Fat	Protein	Carbs	Fiber	Net Carbs
Total:						
Daily Total						

Ketosis: Y/N   Intermittent Fasting: From _____am/pm - To_____am/pm

How'd I do?

Day 12   *Food Tracker*

Daily Target						

Breakfast	Calories	Fat	Protein	Carbs	Fiber	Net Carbs
Total:						

Lunch	Calories	Fat	Protein	Carbs	Fiber	Net Carbs
Total:						

Dinner	Calories	Fat	Protein	Carbs	Fiber	Net Carbs
Total:						

Snacks	Calories	Fat	Protein	Carbs	Fiber	Net Carbs
Total:						

Daily Total						

Ketosis: Y/N   Intermittent Fasting: From ____am/pm - To____am/pm

How'd I do?

Day 13

Date: _____

Daily Target						

Breakfast	Calories	Fat	Protein	Carbs	Fiber	Net Carbs
Total:						

Lunch	Calories	Fat	Protein	Carbs	Fiber	Net Carbs
Total:						

Dinner	Calories	Fat	Protein	Carbs	Fiber	Net Carbs
Total:						

Snacks	Calories	Fat	Protein	Carbs	Fiber	Net Carbs
Total:						

Daily Total						

Ketosis: Y/N   Intermittent Fasting: From _____am/pm - To_____am/pm

How'd I do?

Day 14   Food Tracker

Date: _____
MON TUE WED THU FRI SAT SUN

Daily Target						
Breakfast	Calories	Fat	Protein	Carbs	Fiber	Net Carbs
Total:						
Lunch	Calories	Fat	Protein	Carbs	Fiber	Net Carbs
Total:						
Dinner	Calories	Fat	Protein	Carbs	Fiber	Net Carbs
Total:						
Snacks	Calories	Fat	Protein	Carbs	Fiber	Net Carbs
Total:						
Daily Total						

Ketosis: Y/N   Intermittent Fasting: From _____am/pm - To_____am/pm

How'd I do?

After 14 Days

4"x6"

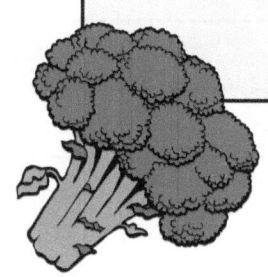

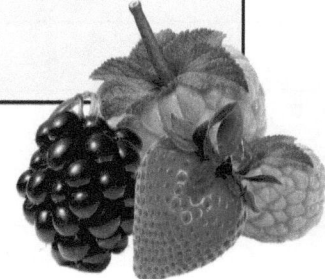

Questions To Ask Myself

Why am I starting the Keto lifestyle?

_____

_____

_____

_____

What's my end goal?

_____

_____

_____

_____

Do I have a weight loss mindset?

_____

_____

_____

_____

Who can I count on for support?

_____

_____

_____

_____

Day 15 – 21

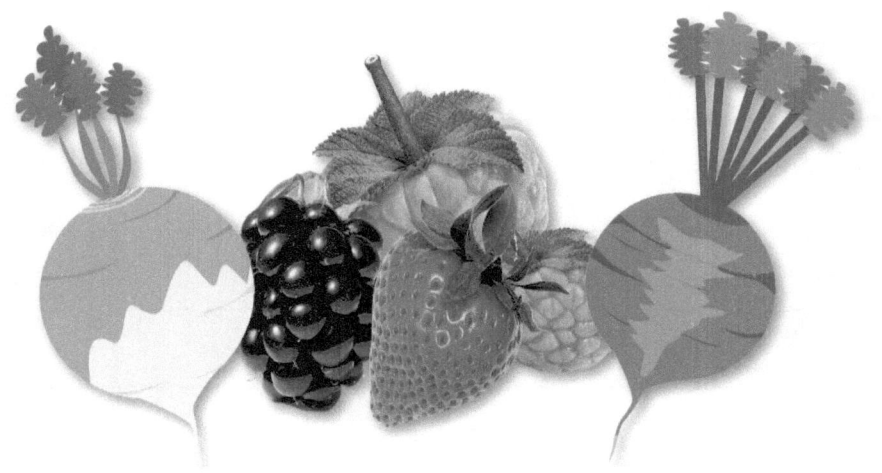

Meal Planner

Day 15 - 21

Day 15	Breakfast: Lunch: Dinner:
Day 16	Breakfast: Lunch: Dinner:
Day 17	Breakfast: Lunch: Dinner:
Day 18	Breakfast: Lunch: Dinner:
Day 19	Breakfast: Lunch: Dinner:
Day 20	Breakfast: Lunch: Dinner:
Day 21	Breakfast: Lunch: Dinner:
Snacks	

Shopping List

MEAT & FISH	DAIRY		VEGETABLES
Bacon	Heavy Cream		Broccoli
Ground Beef	Full Fat Yogurt		Cauliflower
Chicken	Eggs		Cabbage
Cold Cuts	Butter		Cucumber
Pork	Ghee		Eggplant
Lamb	Sour Cream		Bell Pepper
Organ Meats	Cream Cheese		Asparagus
Duck	Full Fat Cheeses		Salad Mix
Steak	**PANTRY**		Spaghetti Squash
Sausage	Pork Rinds		Zuchinni
Shrimp	Almond Milk		Onions
Salmon	Coconut Milk		Garlic
Tuna	Coffee		Celery
FATS & OILS	Himalayan Pink Salt		**FRUITS**
Olive Oil	Mustard		Avocados
Avocado Oil	90% Dark Chocolate		Blueberries
Sesame Oil	Almond Flour		Blackberries
MCT Oil	Coconut Flour		Raspberries
Lard	Bone Broth		Strawberries
Cocoa Butter	Xanthan Gum		Lemons
Coconut Oil	Erythritol		Limes
Nut Butters	Monkfruit		Nuts & Seeds

Shopping List

Day 15 – 21

MEAT & FISH	DAIRY	VEGETABLES
	PANTRY	
FATS & OILS		**FRUITS**

Habit Tracker

HABIT	15	16	17	18	19	20	21	REWARD

Mood Tracker

DAY	MOOD					WHY?
15	🙂	😍	😕	🙁	😣	
16	🙂	😍	😕	🙁	😣	
17	🙂	😍	😕	🙁	😣	
18	🙂	😍	😕	🙁	😣	
19	🙂	😍	😕	🙁	😣	
20	🙂	😍	😕	🙁	😣	
21	🙂	😍	😕	🙁	😣	

 One pound at a time!

Exercise Tracker

Day 15 - 21

Day 15	Day 16	Day 17
Cardio ⚪ Weights⚪	Cardio ⚪ Weights⚪	Cardio ⚪ Weights⚪

Day 18	Day 19	Day 20
Cardio ⚪ Weights⚪	Cardio ⚪ Weights⚪	Cardio ⚪ Weights⚪

Day 21		Day	Calories Burned
		15	
		16	
		17	
		18	
		19	
Cardio ⚪		20	
Weights ⚪		21	

Day 15　Food Tracker

Daily Target						
Breakfast	Calories	Fat	Protein	Carbs	Fiber	Net Carbs
Total:						
Lunch	Calories	Fat	Protein	Carbs	Fiber	Net Carbs
Total:						
Dinner	Calories	Fat	Protein	Carbs	Fiber	Net Carbs
Total:						
Snacks	Calories	Fat	Protein	Carbs	Fiber	Net Carbs
Total:						
Daily Total						

Ketosis: Y/N　Intermittent Fasting: From _____am/pm - To_____am/pm

How'd I do?

Day 16   Food Tracker

Date: _____

MON TUE WED THU FRI SAT SUN

Daily Target						
Breakfast	Calories	Fat	Protein	Carbs	Fiber	Net Carbs
Total:						
Lunch	Calories	Fat	Protein	Carbs	Fiber	Net Carbs
Total:						
Dinner	Calories	Fat	Protein	Carbs	Fiber	Net Carbs
Total:						
Snacks	Calories	Fat	Protein	Carbs	Fiber	Net Carbs
Total:						
Daily Total						

Ketosis: Y/N   Intermittent Fasting: From _____am/pm - To_____am/pm

How'd I do?

_____

_____

_____

_____

_____

_____

_____

_____

_____

_____

_____

_____

_____

_____

_____

_____

_____

_____

Day 17   Food Tracker

Date: _____
MON TUE WED THU FRI SAT SUN

Daily Target						
Breakfast	Calories	Fat	Protein	Carbs	Fiber	Net Carbs
Total:						
Lunch	Calories	Fat	Protein	Carbs	Fiber	Net Carbs
Total:						
Dinner	Calories	Fat	Protein	Carbs	Fiber	Net Carbs
Total:						
Snacks	Calories	Fat	Protein	Carbs	Fiber	Net Carbs
Total:						
Daily Total						

Ketosis: Y/N   Intermittent Fasting: From _____am/pm - To_____am/pm

How'd I do?

Day 18   Food Tracker

Daily Target						
Breakfast	Calories	Fat	Protein	Carbs	Fiber	Net Carbs
Total:						
Lunch	Calories	Fat	Protein	Carbs	Fiber	Net Carbs
Total:						
Dinner	Calories	Fat	Protein	Carbs	Fiber	Net Carbs
Total:						
Snacks	Calories	Fat	Protein	Carbs	Fiber	Net Carbs
Total:						
Daily Total						

Ketosis: Y/N   Intermittent Fasting: From _____am/pm - To_____am/pm

How'd I do?

Day 19   Food Tracker

Date: _____
MON TUE WED THU FRI SAT SUN

Daily Target						

Breakfast	Calories	Fat	Protein	Carbs	Fiber	Net Carbs
Total:						

Lunch	Calories	Fat	Protein	Carbs	Fiber	Net Carbs
Total:						

Dinner	Calories	Fat	Protein	Carbs	Fiber	Net Carbs
Total:						

Snacks	Calories	Fat	Protein	Carbs	Fiber	Net Carbs
Total:						

Daily Total						

Ketosis: Y/N   Intermittent Fasting: From _____am/pm - To_____am/pm

How'd I do?

Day 20   Food Tracker

Daily Target						
Breakfast	Calories	Fat	Protein	Carbs	Fiber	Net Carbs
Total:						
Lunch	Calories	Fat	Protein	Carbs	Fiber	Net Carbs
Total:						
Dinner	Calories	Fat	Protein	Carbs	Fiber	Net Carbs
Total:						
Snacks	Calories	Fat	Protein	Carbs	Fiber	Net Carbs
Total:						
Daily Total						

Ketosis: Y/N   Intermittent Fasting: From _____am/pm - To_____am/pm

How'd I do?

Day 21   Food Tracker

Date: _____
MON TUE WED THU FRI SAT SUN

Daily Target						

Breakfast	Calories	Fat	Protein	Carbs	Fiber	Net Carbs
Total:						

Lunch	Calories	Fat	Protein	Carbs	Fiber	Net Carbs
Total:						

Dinner	Calories	Fat	Protein	Carbs	Fiber	Net Carbs
Total:						

Snacks	Calories	Fat	Protein	Carbs	Fiber	Net Carbs
Total:						

Daily Total						

Ketosis: Y/N   Intermittent Fasting: From _____am/pm - To_____am/pm

How'd I do?

_____

_____

_____

_____

_____

_____

_____

_____

_____

_____

_____

_____

_____

_____

_____

_____

_____

_____

After 21 Days

4"x6"

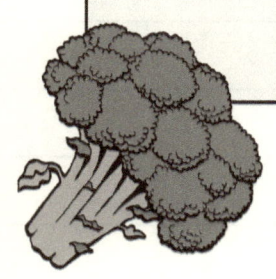
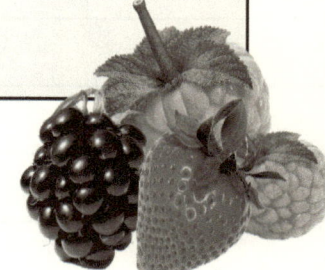

Questions To Ask Myself

Why am I starting the Keto lifestyle?

_____

_____

_____

_____

What's my end goal?

_____

_____

_____

_____

Do I have a weight loss mindset?

_____

_____

_____

_____

Who can I count on for support?

_____

_____

_____

_____

Day 22 - 28

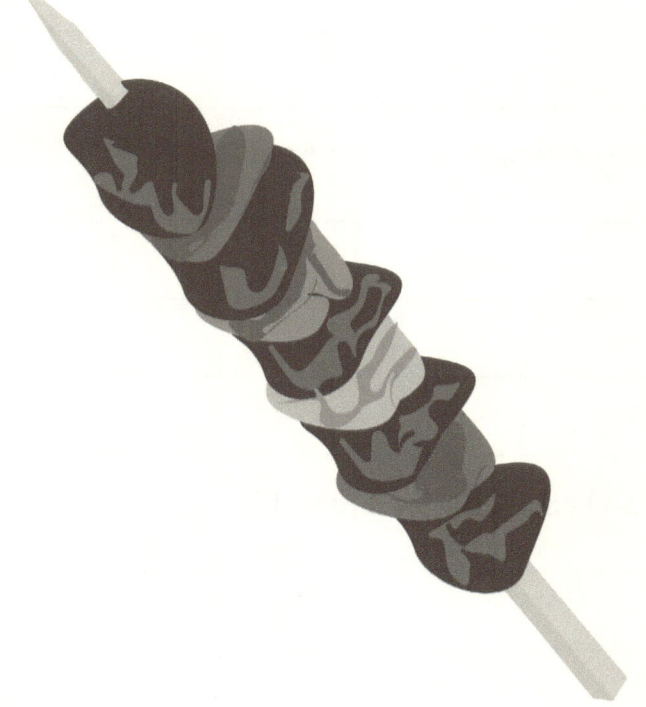

Meal Planner

Day 22	Breakfast: Lunch: Dinner:
Day 23	Breakfast: Lunch: Dinner:
Day 24	Breakfast: Lunch: Dinner:
Day 25	Breakfast: Lunch: Dinner:
Day 26	Breakfast: Lunch: Dinner:
Day 27	Breakfast: Lunch: Dinner:
Day 28	Breakfast: Lunch: Dinner:
Snacks	

Shopping List

Day 22 – 28

MEAT & FISH	DAIRY	VEGETABLES
Bacon	Heavy Cream	Broccoli
Ground Beef	Full Fat Yogurt	Cauliflower
Chicken	Eggs	Cabbage
Cold Cuts	Butter	Cucumber
Pork	Ghee	Eggplant
Lamb	Sour Cream	Bell Pepper
Organ Meats	Cream Cheese	Asparagus
Duck	Full Fat Cheeses	Salad Mix
Steak	**PANTRY**	Spaghetti Squash
Sausage	Pork Rinds	Zuchinni
Shrimp	Almond Milk	Onions
Salmon	Coconut Milk	Garlic
Tuna	Coffee	Celery
FATS & OILS	Himalayan Pink Salt	**FRUITS**
Olive Oil	Mustard	Avocados
Avocado Oil	90% Dark Chocolate	Blueberries
Sesame Oil	Almond Flour	Blackberries
MCT Oil	Coconut Flour	Raspberries
Lard	Bone Broth	Strawberries
Cocoa Butter	Xanthan Gum	Lemons
Coconut Oil	Erythritol	Limes
Nut Butters	Monkfruit	Nuts & Seeds

Shopping List

	MEAT & FISH		DAIRY		VEGETABLES
			PANTRY		
	FATS & OILS				**FRUITS**

Habit Tracker

HABIT	22	23	24	25	26	27	28	REWARD

Mood Tracker

DAY	MOOD					WHY?
22	☺	☻	😧	☹	😨	
23	☺	☻	😧	☹	😨	
24	☺	☻	😧	☹	😨	
25	☺	☻	😧	☹	😨	
26	☺	☻	😧	☹	😨	
27	☺	☻	😧	☹	😨	
28	☺	☻	😧	☹	😨	

 One pound at a time!

Exercise Tracker

Day 22 - 28

Day 22	Day 23	Day 24
Cardio ○ Weights○	Cardio ○ Weights○	Cardio ○ Weights ○

Day 25	Day 26	Day 27
Cardio ○ Weights○	Cardio ○ Weights ○	Cardio ○ Weights ○

Day 28		Day	Calories Burned
		22	
		23	
		24	
		25	
		26	
Cardio ○		27	
Weights ○		28	

Day 22   Food Tracker

Date: _____
MON TUE WED THU FRI SAT SUN

Daily Target						
Breakfast	Calories	Fat	Protein	Carbs	Fiber	Net Carbs
Total:						
Lunch	Calories	Fat	Protein	Carbs	Fiber	Net Carbs
Total:						
Dinner	Calories	Fat	Protein	Carbs	Fiber	Net Carbs
Total:						
Snacks	Calories	Fat	Protein	Carbs	Fiber	Net Carbs
Total:						
Daily Total						

Ketosis: Y/N   Intermittent Fasting: From _____am/pm - To_____am/pm

How'd I do?

Day 23   Food Tracker

Date: _____

Daily Target						
Breakfast	Calories	Fat	Protein	Carbs	Fiber	Net Carbs
Total:						
Lunch	Calories	Fat	Protein	Carbs	Fiber	Net Carbs
Total:						
Dinner	Calories	Fat	Protein	Carbs	Fiber	Net Carbs
Total:						
Snacks	Calories	Fat	Protein	Carbs	Fiber	Net Carbs
Total:						
Daily Total						

Ketosis: Y/N   Intermittent Fasting: From _____am/pm - To_____am/pm

How'd I do?

Day 24 — Food Tracker

Date: _____

MON TUE WED THU FRI SAT SUN

Daily Target						

Breakfast	Calories	Fat	Protein	Carbs	Fiber	Net Carbs
Total:						

Lunch	Calories	Fat	Protein	Carbs	Fiber	Net Carbs
Total:						

Dinner	Calories	Fat	Protein	Carbs	Fiber	Net Carbs
Total:						

Snacks	Calories	Fat	Protein	Carbs	Fiber	Net Carbs
Total:						

Daily Total						

Ketosis: Y/N   Intermittent Fasting: From _____am/pm - To_____am/pm

How'd I do?

Day 25   Food Tracker

Daily Target						
Breakfast	Calories	Fat	Protein	Carbs	Fiber	Net Carbs
Total:						
Lunch	Calories	Fat	Protein	Carbs	Fiber	Net Carbs
Total:						
Dinner	Calories	Fat	Protein	Carbs	Fiber	Net Carbs
Total:						
Snacks	Calories	Fat	Protein	Carbs	Fiber	Net Carbs
Total:						
Daily Total						

Ketosis: Y/N   Intermittent Fasting: From ____am/pm - To____am/pm

How'd I do?

Day 26   Food Tracker

Date: _____
MON TUE WED THU FRI SAT SUN

Daily Target						
Breakfast	Calories	Fat	Protein	Carbs	Fiber	Net Carbs
Total:						
Lunch	Calories	Fat	Protein	Carbs	Fiber	Net Carbs
Total:						
Dinner	Calories	Fat	Protein	Carbs	Fiber	Net Carbs
Total:						
Snacks	Calories	Fat	Protein	Carbs	Fiber	Net Carbs
Total:						
Daily Total						

Ketosis: Y/N   Intermittent Fasting: From _____am/pm - To_____am/pm

How'd I do?

Day 27 Food Tracker

Daily Target						

Breakfast	Calories	Fat	Protein	Carbs	Fiber	Net Carbs
Total:						

Lunch	Calories	Fat	Protein	Carbs	Fiber	Net Carbs
Total:						

Dinner	Calories	Fat	Protein	Carbs	Fiber	Net Carbs
Total:						

Snacks	Calories	Fat	Protein	Carbs	Fiber	Net Carbs
Total:						

Daily Total						

Ketosis: Y/N   Intermittent Fasting: From _____am/pm - To_____am/pm

How'd I do?

Day 28   Food Tracker

Date: _____
MON TUE WED THU FRI SAT SUN

Daily Target						

Breakfast	Calories	Fat	Protein	Carbs	Fiber	Net Carbs
Total:						

Lunch	Calories	Fat	Protein	Carbs	Fiber	Net Carbs
Total:						

Dinner	Calories	Fat	Protein	Carbs	Fiber	Net Carbs
Total:						

Snacks	Calories	Fat	Protein	Carbs	Fiber	Net Carbs
Total:						

Daily Total						

Ketosis: Y/N   Intermittent Fasting: From _____am/pm - To_____am/pm

How'd I do?

After 28 Days

4"x6"

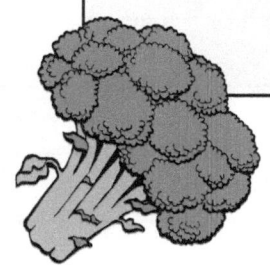
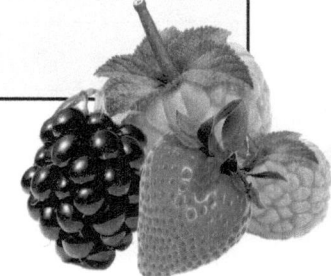

Questions To Ask Yourself

Will I continue with this way of eating? Why or why not?

_____

_____

_____

_____

Can I do this alone or do I need more support?

_____

_____

_____

_____

Even if I reach my goal I will stick to Keto. True or False?

_____

_____

_____

_____

I would recommend the Keto lifestyle to friends & family?

_____

_____

_____

_____

I Can

&

I Did !

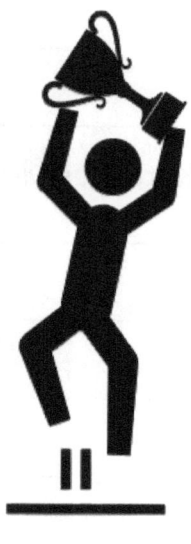

Keto

Recipes

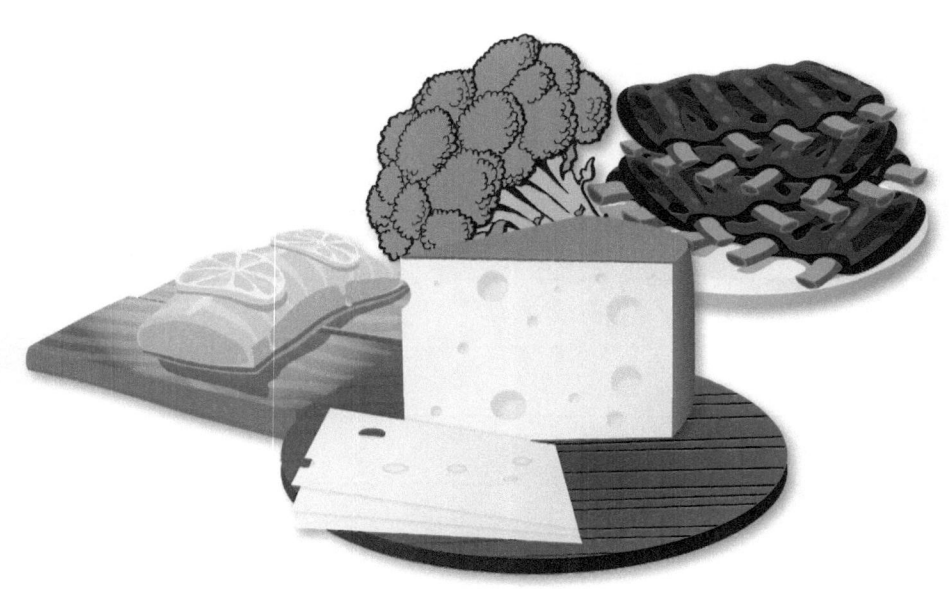

Recipe: _____

Prep Time [   ] Cook Time [   ] Servings [   ] Difficulty [   ]

Ingredients

_____

_____

_____

_____

_____

_____

Directions

_____

_____

_____

_____

_____

_____

_____

_____

_____

_____

Protein [   ] Fat [   ] Carbs [   ] Fiber [   ] Calories [   ]

Recipe: _____

Prep Time [   ] Cook Time [   ] Servings [   ] Difficulty [   ]

Ingredients

_____

_____

_____

_____

_____

_____

Directions

_____

_____

_____

_____

_____

_____

_____

_____

_____

_____

_____

Protein [   ] Fat [   ] Carbs [   ] Fiber [   ] Calories [   ]

Recipe: _____

Prep Time [   ] Cook Time [   ] Servings [   ] Difficulty [   ]

Ingredients

_____

_____

_____

_____

_____

_____

Directions

_____

_____

_____

_____

_____

_____

_____

_____

_____

Protein [   ] Fat [   ] Carbs [   ] Fiber [   ] Calories [   ]

Recipe: _____

Prep Time [   ] Cook Time [   ] Servings [   ] Difficulty [   ]

Ingredients

_____

_____

_____

_____

_____

_____

Directions

_____

_____

_____

_____

_____

_____

_____

_____

_____

_____

Protein [   ] Fat [   ] Carbs [   ] Fiber [   ] Calories [   ]

Recipe: _____

Prep Time [　　] Cook Time [　　] Servings [　　] Difficulty [　　]

Ingredients

_____

_____

_____

_____

_____

_____

Directions

_____

_____

_____

_____

_____

_____

_____

_____

_____

_____

Protein [　　] Fat [　　] Carbs [　　] Fiber [　　] Calories [　　]

Recipe: _____

Prep Time [   ] Cook Time [   ] Servings [   ] Difficulty [   ]

Ingredients

_____

_____

_____

_____

_____

_____

Directions

_____

_____

_____

_____

_____

_____

_____

_____

_____

_____

Protein [   ] Fat [   ] Carbs [   ] Fiber [   ] Calories [   ]

Recipe: _____

Prep Time [   ] Cook Time [   ] Servings [   ] Difficulty [   ]

Ingredients

_____

_____

_____

_____

_____

_____

Directions

_____

_____

_____

_____

_____

_____

_____

_____

_____

_____

Protein [   ] Fat [   ] Carbs [   ] Fiber [   ] Calories [   ]

Recipe: _____

Prep Time [   ] Cook Time [   ] Servings [   ] Difficulty [   ]

Ingredients

_____

_____

_____

_____

_____

_____

Directions

_____

_____

_____

_____

_____

_____

_____

_____

_____

_____

Protein [   ] Fat [   ] Carbs [   ] Fiber [   ] Calories [   ]

Recipe: _____

Prep Time [   ] Cook Time [   ] Servings [   ] Difficulty [   ]

Ingredients

_____

_____

_____

_____

_____

_____

_____

Directions

_____

_____

_____

_____

_____

_____

_____

_____

_____

_____

_____

Protein [   ] Fat [   ] Carbs [   ] Fiber [   ] Calories [   ]

Recipe: _____

Prep Time [   ] Cook Time [   ] Servings [   ] Difficulty [   ]

Ingredients

_____

_____

_____

_____

_____

_____

Directions

_____

_____

_____

_____

_____

_____

_____

_____

_____

_____

_____

Protein [   ] Fat [   ] Carbs [   ] Fiber [   ] Calories [   ]

Recipe: _____

Prep Time [   ] Cook Time [   ] Servings [   ] Difficulty [   ]

Ingredients

_____

_____

_____

_____

_____

_____

Directions

_____

_____

_____

_____

_____

_____

_____

_____

_____

_____

Protein [   ] Fat [   ] Carbs [   ] Fiber [   ] Calories [   ]

Recipe: _____

Prep Time [   ] Cook Time [   ] Servings [   ] Difficulty [   ]

Ingredients

_____

_____

_____

_____

_____

_____

Directions

_____

_____

_____

_____

_____

_____

_____

_____

_____

_____

_____

Protein [   ] Fat [   ] Carbs [   ] Fiber [   ] Calories [   ]

Recipe: _____

Prep Time [   ] Cook Time [   ] Servings [   ] Difficulty [   ]

Ingredients

_____

_____

_____

_____

_____

_____

Directions

_____

_____

_____

_____

_____

_____

_____

_____

_____

_____

_____

Protein [   ] Fat [   ] Carbs [   ] Fiber [   ] Calories [   ]

Recipe: _____

Prep Time [   ] Cook Time [   ] Servings [   ] Difficulty [   ]

Ingredients

_____

_____

_____

_____

_____

_____

Directions

_____

_____

_____

_____

_____

_____

_____

_____

_____

_____

_____

Protein [   ] Fat [   ] Carbs [   ] Fiber [   ] Calories [   ]

Recipe: _____

Prep Time [   ] Cook Time [   ] Servings [   ] Difficulty [   ]

Ingredients

_____

_____

_____

_____

_____

_____

Directions

_____

_____

_____

_____

_____

_____

_____

_____

_____

_____

Protein [   ] Fat [   ] Carbs [   ] Fiber [   ] Calories [   ]

Recipe: _____

Prep Time [   ] Cook Time [   ] Servings [   ] Difficulty [   ]

Ingredients

_____

_____

_____

_____

_____

_____

_____

Directions

_____

_____

_____

_____

_____

_____

_____

_____

_____

_____

_____

_____

Protein [   ] Fat [   ] Carbs [   ] Fiber [   ] Calories [   ]

Recipe: _____

Prep Time [   ] Cook Time [   ] Servings [   ] Difficulty [   ]

Ingredients

_____

_____

_____

_____

_____

_____

_____

Directions

_____

_____

_____

_____

_____

_____

_____

_____

_____

_____

_____

Protein [   ] Fat [   ] Carbs [   ] Fiber [   ] Calories [   ]

Recipe: _____

Prep Time [   ] Cook Time [   ] Servings [   ] Difficulty [   ]

Ingredients

_____

_____

_____

_____

_____

_____

Directions

_____

_____

_____

_____

_____

_____

_____

_____

_____

_____

Protein [   ] Fat [   ] Carbs [   ] Fiber [   ] Calories [   ]

Recipe: _____

Prep Time [   ] Cook Time [   ] Servings [   ] Difficulty [   ]

Ingredients

_____

_____

_____

_____

_____

_____

Directions

_____

_____

_____

_____

_____

_____

_____

_____

_____

_____

Protein [   ] Fat [   ] Carbs [   ] Fiber [   ] Calories [   ]

Recipe: _____

Prep Time [   ] Cook Time [   ] Servings [   ] Difficulty [   ]

Ingredients

_____

_____

_____

_____

_____

_____

Directions

_____

_____

_____

_____

_____

_____

_____

_____

_____

_____

_____

Protein [   ] Fat [   ] Carbs [   ] Fiber [   ] Calories [   ]

Recipe: _____

Prep Time [   ] Cook Time [   ] Servings [   ] Difficulty [   ]

Ingredients

_____

_____

_____

_____

_____

_____

_____

Directions

_____

_____

_____

_____

_____

_____

_____

_____

_____

_____

_____

Protein [   ] Fat [   ] Carbs [   ] Fiber [   ] Calories [   ]

Recipe: _____

Prep Time [   ] Cook Time [   ] Servings [   ] Difficulty [   ]

Ingredients

_____

_____

_____

_____

_____

_____

_____

Directions

_____

_____

_____

_____

_____

_____

_____

_____

_____

_____

_____

Protein [   ] Fat [   ] Carbs [   ] Fiber [   ] Calories [   ]

Recipe: _____

Prep Time [   ] Cook Time [   ] Servings [   ] Difficulty [   ]

Ingredients

_____

_____

_____

_____

_____

_____

Directions

_____

_____

_____

_____

_____

_____

_____

_____

_____

_____

Protein [   ] Fat [   ] Carbs [   ] Fiber [   ] Calories [   ]

Recipe: _____

Prep Time [   ] Cook Time [   ] Servings [   ] Difficulty [   ]

Ingredients

_____

_____

_____

_____

_____

_____

_____

Directions

_____

_____

_____

_____

_____

_____

_____

_____

_____

_____

_____

Protein [   ] Fat [   ] Carbs [   ] Fiber [   ] Calories [   ]

Recipe: _____

Prep Time [   ] Cook Time [   ] Servings [   ] Difficulty [   ]

Ingredients

_____

_____

_____

_____

_____

_____

Directions

_____

_____

_____

_____

_____

_____

_____

_____

_____

_____

_____

Protein [   ] Fat [   ] Carbs [   ] Fiber [   ] Calories [   ]

Recipe: _____

Prep Time [   ] Cook Time [   ] Servings [   ] Difficulty [   ]

Ingredients

_____

_____

_____

_____

_____

_____

_____

Directions

_____

_____

_____

_____

_____

_____

_____

_____

_____

_____

Protein [   ] Fat [   ] Carbs [   ] Fiber [   ] Calories [   ]

Recipe: _____

Prep Time [   ] Cook Time [   ] Servings [   ] Difficulty [   ]

Ingredients

_____

_____

_____

_____

_____

_____

Directions

_____

_____

_____

_____

_____

_____

_____

_____

_____

_____

_____

_____

Protein [   ] Fat [   ] Carbs [   ] Fiber [   ] Calories [   ]

Recipe: _____

Prep Time [   ] Cook Time [   ] Servings [   ] Difficulty [   ]

Ingredients

_____

_____

_____

_____

_____

_____

Directions

_____

_____

_____

_____

_____

_____

_____

_____

_____

_____

Protein [   ] Fat [   ] Carbs [   ] Fiber [   ] Calories [   ]

Recipe: _____

Prep Time [   ] Cook Time [   ] Servings [   ] Difficulty [   ]

Ingredients

_____

_____

_____

_____

_____

_____

Directions

_____

_____

_____

_____

_____

_____

_____

_____

_____

_____

Protein [   ] Fat [   ] Carbs [   ] Fiber [   ] Calories [   ]

Recipe: _____

Prep Time [   ] Cook Time [   ] Servings [   ] Difficulty [   ]

Ingredients

_____

_____

_____

_____

_____

_____

_____

Directions

_____

_____

_____

_____

_____

_____

_____

_____

_____

_____

_____

Protein [   ] Fat [   ] Carbs [   ] Fiber [   ] Calories [   ]

Recipe: _____

Prep Time [   ] Cook Time [   ] Servings [   ] Difficulty [   ]

Ingredients

_____

_____

_____

_____

_____

_____

_____

Directions

_____

_____

_____

_____

_____

_____

_____

_____

_____

_____

_____

Protein [   ] Fat [   ] Carbs [   ] Fiber [   ] Calories [   ]

Recipe: _____

Prep Time [　　] Cook Time [　　] Servings [　　] Difficulty [　　]

Ingredients

_____

_____

_____

_____

_____

_____

Directions

_____

_____

_____

_____

_____

_____

_____

_____

_____

_____

Protein [　　] Fat [　　] Carbs [　　] Fiber [　　] Calories [　　]

Recipe: _____

Prep Time [   ] Cook Time [   ] Servings [   ] Difficulty [   ]

Ingredients

_____

_____

_____

_____

_____

_____

_____

Directions

_____

_____

_____

_____

_____

_____

_____

_____

_____

_____

_____

Protein [   ] Fat [   ] Carbs [   ] Fiber [   ] Calories [   ]

Recipe: _____

Prep Time [   ] Cook Time [   ] Servings [   ] Difficulty [   ]

Ingredients

_____

_____

_____

_____

_____

_____

Directions

_____

_____

_____

_____

_____

_____

_____

_____

_____

Protein [   ] Fat [   ] Carbs [   ] Fiber [   ] Calories [   ]

Recipe: _____

Prep Time [   ] Cook Time [   ] Servings [   ] Difficulty [   ]

Ingredients

_____

_____

_____

_____

_____

_____

Directions

_____

_____

_____

_____

_____

_____

_____

_____

_____

_____

Protein [   ] Fat [   ] Carbs [   ] Fiber [   ] Calories [   ]

Recipe: _____

Prep Time [   ] Cook Time [   ] Servings [   ] Difficulty [   ]

Ingredients

_____

_____

_____

_____

_____

_____

_____

Directions

_____

_____

_____

_____

_____

_____

_____

_____

_____

_____

_____

Protein [   ] Fat [   ] Carbs [   ] Fiber [   ] Calories [   ]

Recipe: _____

Prep Time [   ] Cook Time [   ] Servings [   ] Difficulty [   ]

Ingredients

_____

_____

_____

_____

_____

_____

Directions

_____

_____

_____

_____

_____

_____

_____

_____

_____

_____

_____

Protein [   ] Fat [   ] Carbs [   ] Fiber [   ] Calories [   ]

Recipe: _____

Prep Time [   ] Cook Time [   ] Servings [   ] Difficulty [   ]

Ingredients

_____

_____

_____

_____

_____

Directions

_____

_____

_____

_____

_____

_____

_____

_____

_____

Protein [   ] Fat [   ] Carbs [   ] Fiber [   ] Calories [   ]

Recipe: _____

Prep Time [   ] Cook Time [   ] Servings [   ] Difficulty [   ]

Ingredients

_____

_____

_____

_____

_____

_____

Directions

_____

_____

_____

_____

_____

_____

_____

_____

_____

_____

Protein [   ] Fat [   ] Carbs [   ] Fiber [   ] Calories [   ]

Recipe: _____

Prep Time [   ] Cook Time [   ] Servings [   ] Difficulty [   ]

Ingredients

_____

_____

_____

_____

_____

_____

Directions

_____

_____

_____

_____

_____

_____

_____

_____

_____

_____

Protein [   ] Fat [   ] Carbs [   ] Fiber [   ] Calories [   ]

Recipe: _____

Prep Time [   ] Cook Time [   ] Servings [   ] Difficulty [   ]

Ingredients

_____

_____

_____

_____

_____

_____

Directions

_____

_____

_____

_____

_____

_____

_____

_____

_____

_____

_____

_____

Protein [   ] Fat [   ] Carbs [   ] Fiber [   ] Calories [   ]